FERTILITY BOOSTING FOODS

DISCLAIMER

TABLE OF CONTENT

INTRODUCTION

Although it's important to keep in mind that every person's diet will affect fertility differently, several foods are known to have fertility-enhancing properties. Despite the fact that they might not always lead to conception, these nutrients can nevertheless help with general reproductive health. Here are a few foods that have a history of supporting increased fertility.

LEAFY GREEN: Vegetables are an excellent addition to a healthy diet, including for promoting reproductive health. Here are some benefits that they offer:

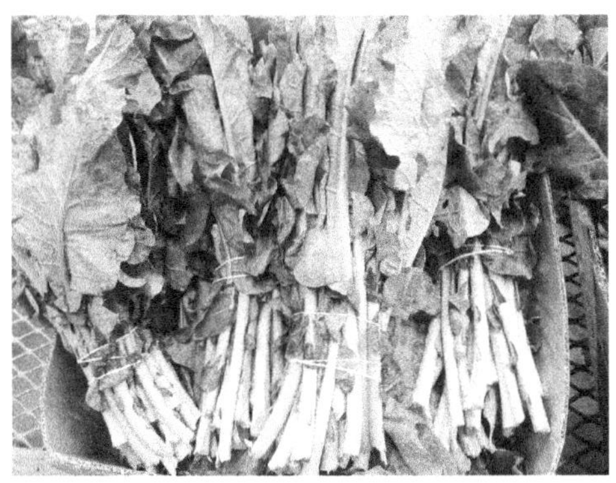

Leafy greens like spinach, kale, Swiss chard, and arugula are rich in folate (vitamin B9). For fetal growth and fertility, folate is crucial. Inadequate folate consumption is linked to neonatal neural tube defects.

Among the many antioxidants that are present in large quantities in these plants are vitamin C, vitamin E, and beta-carotene. Free radicals have a negative effect on reproductive health and can damage cells. Cells are better protected from this harm by antioxidants.

Iron: A healthy uterus needs the mineral iron, which is present in leafy greens. Iron aids in the correct blood flow and oxygen delivery that the reproductive organs require.

DIETARY FIBER, Which is abundant in leafy greens, helps manage insulin levels and maintain a healthy weight. Fertility can benefit from effective insulin control and weight management.

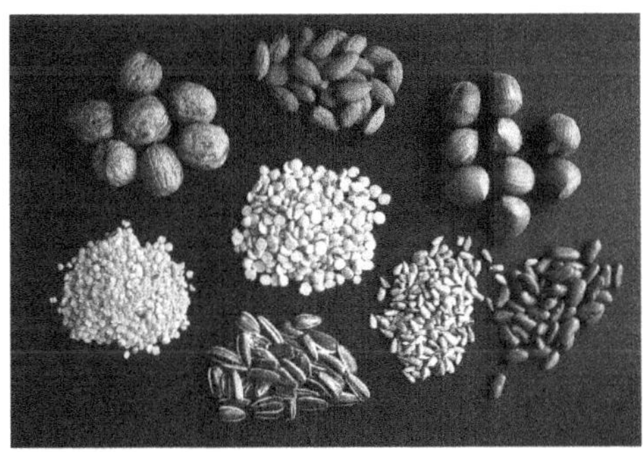

Although leafy greens frequently have little calories, they are also a good source of vitamins A, C, and K as well as minerals like calcium and magnesium. These nutrients support overall wellness, which encompasses reproductive health.

Consider both cooked and raw varieties of leafy greens when incorporating them into your diet. They complement steamed, stir-fried, salad, smoothie, and other dishes wonderfully. Don't forget to thoroughly wash them before eating them.

It's important to keep in mind that a healthy diet is just one of several things that can enhance reproductive health. If you're having trouble getting pregnant, you should speak with a medical expert to get a full evaluation and personalized advice.

A healthy diet must include whole grains because they have several benefits for sexual and reproductive health. The following list of benefits for including whole grains:

WHOLE GRAINS: Are a good source of dietary fiber, which promotes digestive health and aids with blood sugar regulation. Controlling blood sugar can help keep hormone levels in check, especially those that affect reproduction.

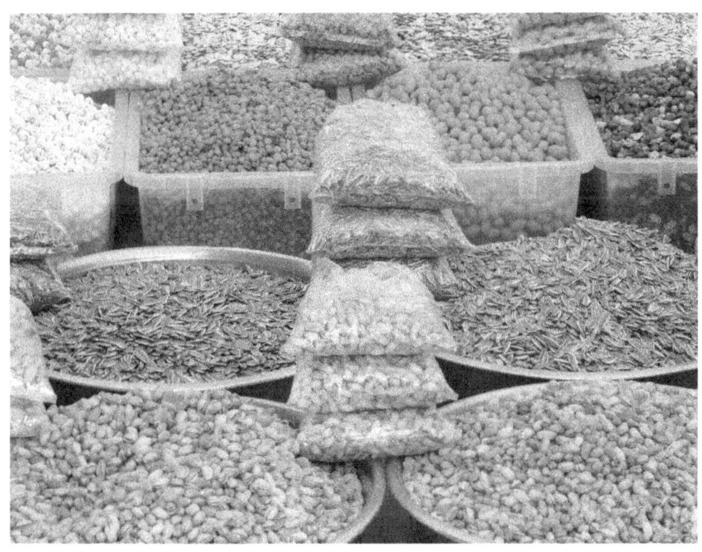

Complex carbs, which release energy gradually over time, are found in whole grains. They can help prevent blood sugar fluctuations, which can be bad for the balance of hormones and reproductive health.

Whole grains are a great source of vitamins and minerals, such as vitamin E, magnesium, and selenium, in addition to B vitamins (such as folate, thiamin, and niacin). These vitamins and minerals support healthy hormone production and reproduction.

Lower Glycemic Index: Compared to refined grains, whole grains frequently have a lower glycemic index. Foods with a low glycemic index slowly release glucose into the blood, preventing sharp rises in blood sugar levels. Since it maintains constant insulin levels, this is helpful for reproductive health.

Reduced Inflammation: Whole grains contain phytonutrients and antioxidants that may help to reduce inflammation in the body. Because chronic inflammation has been demonstrated to negatively affect reproductive health, eating anti-inflammatory foods like whole grains may be beneficial.

Pick whole grains for your diet, such as quinoa, brown rice, oats, whole wheat, barley, and buckwheat. These go well with soups, salads, and grain bowls. They can also be served as a side dish.

Remember that a diversified diet that is adequate in nutrient-dense foods and is balanced overall is essential for reproductive health. If you have specific inquiries about fertility or reproductive health, speak with a healthcare professional for personalized guidance.

FATTENING FISH: Enhance a healthy diet by encouraging, among other things, reproductive health. The advantages of having fatty fish in your diet include the following:

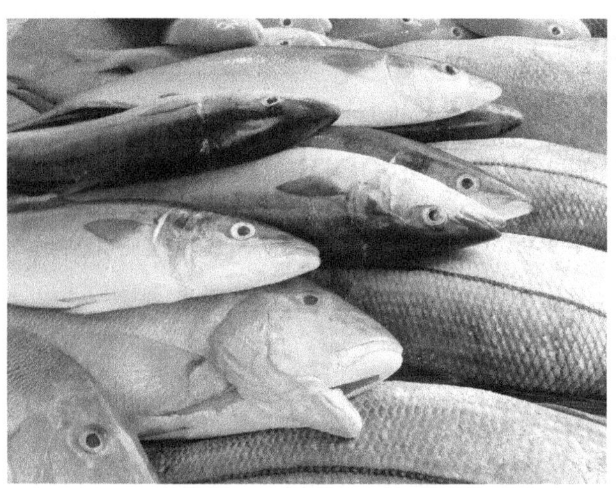

Two critical omega-3 fatty acids, EPA (eicosapentaenoic acid) and DHA (docosahexaenoic acid), are prevalent in fatty fish including salmon, mackerel, sardines, and trout. These omega-3 fatty acids have been associated with improved fertility and reproductive health. They support healthy sperm and egg development, reduce inflammation, and maintain hormone levels.

Hormonal Harmony: The body's hormonal harmony can be supported by omega-3 fatty acids, which are found in fatty fish. They aid in the production of prostaglandins, hormone-like substances crucial to several reproductive processes, including ovulation.

Anti-Inflammatory Properties: Fatty fish contains anti-inflammatory compounds that may help to reduce inflammation in the body.
Because persistent inflammation can have negative effects on reproductive health, eating anti-inflammatory foods like fatty fish may be beneficial.

Salmon and other fatty fish are excellent sources of vitamin D. Vitamin D has an impact on both hormone control and general reproductive health.

An important nutrient for both general health and reproduction, high-quality protein is also found in abundance in fatty fish.
Selenium, vitamin B12, and zinc are among the essential nutrients they provide, all of which assist hormone production and reproductive health.

When including fatty fish in your diet, it is suggested to choose wild-caught fish over farm-raised fish to minimize potential exposure to pollutants. Try to include fatty fish in your meals at least twice a week.

Although eating a balanced diet can aid with reproductive health, this is only one factor.
If you're having trouble getting pregnant, you should speak with a medical expert to get a full evaluation and personalized advice.

BERRIES

Berries are a delicious and healthy fruit that offer several benefits for reproductive health. Berries provide the following advantages when added to your diet:

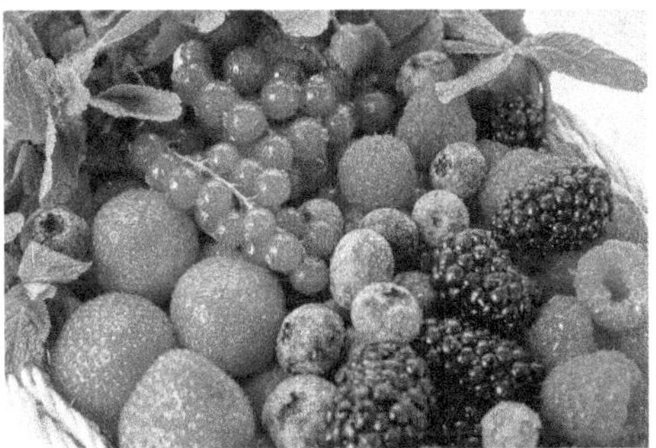

Berry Power: Berries including blueberries, strawberries, raspberries, and blackberries are high in antioxidants. Vitamin C, anthocyanins, and flavonoids are some examples of these anti-oxidants. They help to stop oxidative stress and cell damage in the body. By protecting the sperm and eggs, they help to maintain the reproductive system's overall health.

Better Ovulation: Some studies suggest that eating berries frequently may aid in ovulation.
Strong antioxidants found in berries may help regulate reproductive hormone levels and promote regular ovulation.

Fruits rich in nutrients like berries provide essential vitamins and minerals. They include a lot of vitamins and minerals as well. Vitamin C, which is essential for hormone synthesis and reproduction, is particularly abundant in them. Berries also contain folate, which is crucial for a healthy prenatal development and reducing the risk of neural tube defects.

Berries are a great source of dietary fiber, which supports good digestion and helps regulate blood sugar levels. Controlling blood sugar is crucial for healthy hormone balance and reproduction.

Low in Calories: Berries provide little calories but a potent flavor. In place of sugary snacks, which can cause hormonal imbalances and weight gain, they can be a delightful and healthy option.

Berries can be consumed as a snack or added to desserts, smoothies, cereal, salads, and yogurt. Try to include a variety of berries in your diet to benefit from the many nutrients that berries have to offer.

Remember that preserving reproductive health involves many different factors, including a healthy diet. If you have specific concerns or are experiencing problems conceiving, speak with a healthcare professional for personalized guidance and assistance.

LEGUMES

A few of the very nutrient-dense legumes that can support reproductive health include beans, lentils, chickpeas, and peas. The advantages of adding legumes in your diet are as follows:

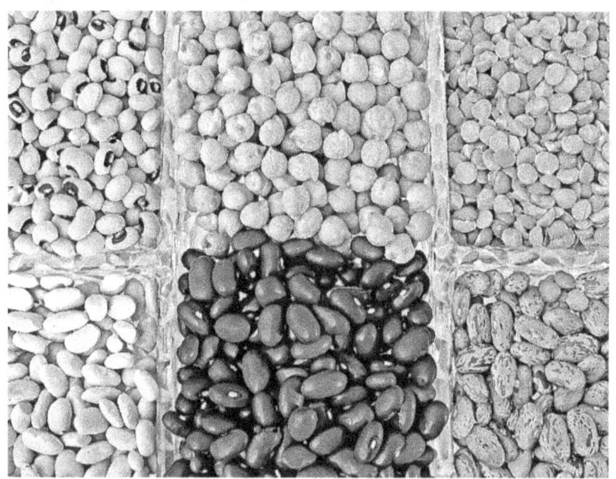

Plant-based protein: A fantastic source of plant-based protein is legumes. Protein is necessary for the development of healthy sperm and eggs as well as for the production of reproductive hormones. For sustaining healthy reproductive health, it's imperative to consume adequate protein daily.

Due to the high dietary fiber content of legumes, a healthy digestive system and blood sugar levels are supported. Controlling blood sugar levels can enhance hormonal balance and reproductive health.

Complex carbohydrates, which are digested more gradually than simple carbohydrates, are present in legumes.
As a result, insulin levels are maintained and energy is released gradually. A healthy balance of insulin levels is beneficial for the reproductive system.

In addition to other B vitamins, legumes are a good source of folate (vitamin B9). Folate is crucial for reproductive health because it supports proper embryonic development and reduces the risk of neural tube defects. B vitamins also have an impact on hormone production and general reproductive health.

Minerals: Legumes include significant amounts of iron, magnesium, and zinc. Iron is necessary for healthy blood flow, which is essential for reproductive organs. Magnesium and zinc play a role in hormone regulation and reproductive health in general.

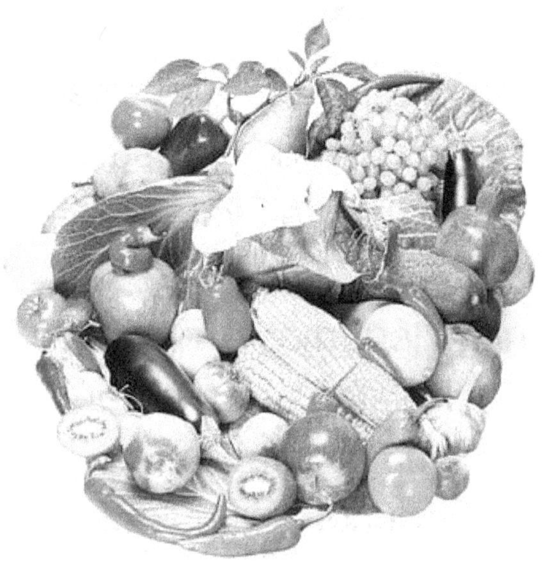

One simple approach to include beans in your diet is to simply add them to salads, soups, stews, or side dishes. Furthermore, you might use them as the base for vegan recipes like lentil or bean curries.

While eating healthy is beneficial for reproductive health, it's crucial to keep in mind that this is just one of several factors. If you have specific queries or are experiencing problems conceiving, it is advisable to speak with a healthcare professional for personalized guidance and support.

HEALTHY FATS: Are necessary for many biological functions and are essential for a balanced diet. They provide energy, encourage cell growth, protect organs, aid in vitamin absorption, and encourage the creation of hormones. Here are some examples of healthy fats:

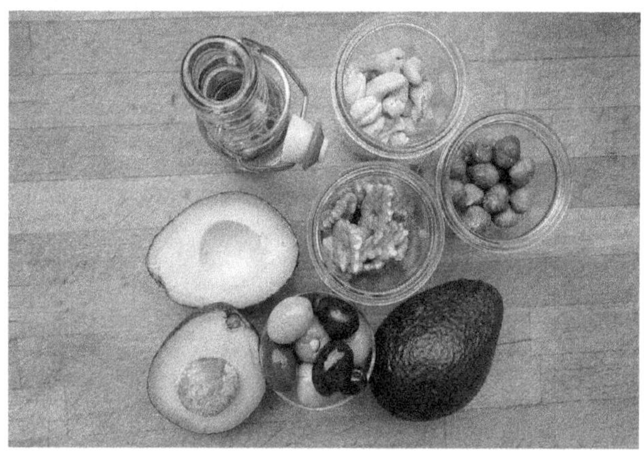

Avocados: Due to their high content of monounsaturated fatty acids, avocados can help reduce bad cholesterol levels as well as the risk of heart disease. They also contain potassium, fiber, and a range of vitamins and minerals.

Nuts and seeds: Almonds, walnuts, chia seeds, flaxseeds, and hemp seeds are fantastic sources of good fats. Additionally, they are a great source of vitamins, minerals, and omega-3 fatty acids, including magnesium and vitamin E.

Monounsaturated fatty acids are abundant in olive oil, which is a staple of the Mediterranean diet. It has been associated to numerous health benefits, including reduced inflammation and improved heart function.

Fish high in omega-3 fatty acids include sardines, mackerel, trout, salmon, and mackerel. These fats have positive effects on the heart, the brain, and have anti-inflammatory properties.

Coconut oil contains medium-chain triglycerides (MCTs), which are easily absorbed and used as a source of energy. Coconut oil should only be used sparingly because of how much saturated fat it contains.

Seeds: Monounsaturated and polyunsaturated fats, which are excellent for you, are abundant in sunflower and pumpkin seeds. Additionally, they provide crucial minerals including magnesium and zinc.

Natural nut butters, such as almond or peanut butter, can be an excellent source of fats when consumed in moderation. Look for products without added sweeteners or hydrogenated oils.

Dark chocolate: With a high cocoa content (70%) contains monounsaturated fats and the antioxidant chemical class known as flavanols. Your sweet tooth may be better satisfied by choosing this choice.

Despite the fact that they do include some saturated fats, eggs are a healthy source of monounsaturated and polyunsaturated fats. They contain a ton of high-quality protein components, vitamins, and minerals.

Dairy: Full-fat dairy products, such as yogurt, cheese, and milk, provide healthy fats. However, it's important to choose items without added sugars and consume them in moderation.

When including healthy fats in your diet, keep in mind that they are high in calories and should be consumed in moderation. Maintaining a balanced diet with a variety of nutrient-rich foods is essential to promoting general health and wellbeing.

BEANS AND LENTILS: These very nutrient-dense legumes are an excellent source of good fats and have a variety of additional health benefits. The main selling feature of these foods is their high protein and fiber content, but they also include beneficial fats that support overall wellbeing. Below are further details about the healthy fats found in beans and lentils.

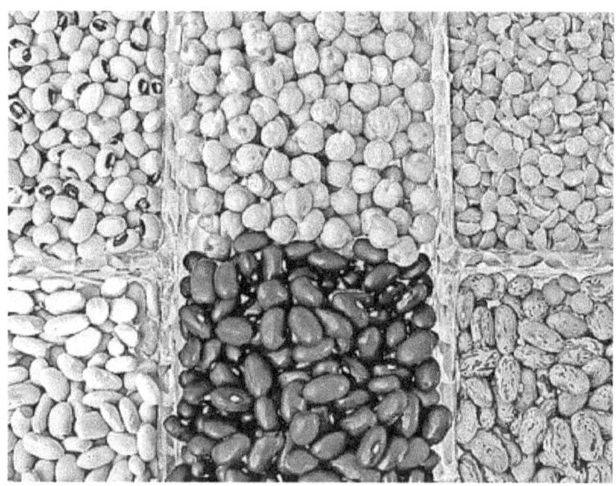

The polyunsaturated fats in beans and lentils include omega-3 and omega-6 fatty acids. These fats are regarded as required because the body cannot produce them on its own and must obtain them from the food.

Omega-3 fatty acids contain anti-inflammatory properties, are essential for heart health, and support cognitive function while omega-6 fatty acids support growth and development.

MONOUNSATURATED FATS, which have been connected to a range of health benefits, are also present in beans and lentils. These fats can increase blood cholesterol levels, support insulin sensitivity, and reduce the risk of heart disease.

Despite the fact that fiber is not a fat in and of itself, beans and lentils contain significant amounts of it. It is necessary for maintaining blood sugar regulation, promoting satiety, and protecting the digestive system's health. Foods high in fiber can help with weight management and may reduce the risk of contracting several chronic illnesses, such as diabetes, heart disease, and some malignancies.

Eating beans and lentils can help you include healthy fats and other essential nutrients in your diet. They are versatile ingredients that may be used into a variety of cuisines, such as salads, sides, soups, and stews. Because they are frequently affordable and have a lengthy shelf life, legumes are a sensible and practical choice for a wholesome diet.

Remind yourself to fully cook beans and lentils to improve digestion and reduce anti-nutrients. They can be cleaned up by soaking and washing them before cooking to help get rid of some of the contaminants that could lead to digestive discomfort.

Before making any dietary decisions, it is always advisable to contact with a healthcare provider or a qualified dietitian in order to get personalized advice based on your particular health needs and goals.

CONCLUSION

In conclusion, adding items that promote fertility to your diet can be helpful for single people or couples who are trying to get pregnant. These meals can enhance general reproductive health and improve the likelihood of a successful conception, even if they cannot guarantee pregnancy.